Bushcraft Book

The ultimate field guide to the art Of Wilderness survival. Essential Skills, Tactics, Techniques, Technologies for Uncertain World.

Dedication

Thank you for buying my book.

I wrote it for you, dear reader; I dedicate it to you, whoever you are and whatever your experience with the art of survival is.

As I tried to write a book about survival, I came to the conclusion that I should give as much knowledge as possible. At the same time, I came to the conclusion that what I want to communicate to you is only the tip of the iceberg. After all, it is not possible to include all my life experiences on several dozen pages. Especially since people's experiences are very different, each of us is different in origin, in nationality.

We live in different countries, in different climates, and it is not possible to write a survival manual that would be suitable for all of us. That is why I decided to share with you the knowledge that can be used in most cases. I tried it to be as universal as it is possible. At the same time, being aware that I will not exhaust the topic and that something can always happen that is characteristic of a particular climate zone. You will agree for sure that other challenges will be faced when you find yourself in the Caucasus mountains in winter, others when you wander in the Mississippi or Amazon basin, and others when you set up a camp somewhere near the Arctic Circle. Extremely different climatic and terrain conditions often lead to extremely different solutions. So what you will find in this book will be some universal rules that you will be able to apply everywhere. Provided that you should approach them creatively, making the right modifications, appropriate to the conditions you live in.

At the same time, I would like you to treat my book as an introduction to the art of survival. I would like to inspire you to search for information on your own and develop by regularly expanding the dictionary of equivalent terms and gaining experience in the field.

I wish you a pleasant reading; I hope that my modest book will make you want to learn new things and that over time you will become confident that you will be able to cope in any conditions and in any survival situation.

Ryan Jones

Preface

Today, we are surrounded by facilities that are intended by their creators to make life easier and help in various situations. From knife and fork to quantum computers, we have technology that makes our lives easier and more comfortable. We no longer need horses or dog sleds to move from place to place. Cities and villages are connected by highways, which we travel through in comfortable, air-conditioned cars with automatic transmission, cruise control, and high-quality music from the speakers, making our journey more pleasant. It is obvious that this was not always the case. Until 200 years ago, we set off on a journey without counting that it would take place in comfortable conditions. We knew that we would have to sleep under the open sky, that we would only be able to warm ourselves by the fire that we would make on our own, and it was not uncommon that we had to get the food ourselves. We had to be inventive and creative to survive.

With the passing of decades and technological progress, our lifestyle has changed. Food, shelter, and transportation methods have now reached a level unattainable for our ancestors. We live today in times that enable us to pursue personal goals without having to leave our comfort zone. In addition to the obvious benefits of modern reality, we sometimes ask ourselves a question:

How will I cope with the challenges and dangers if all these conveniences and achievements of civilization are missing overnight?

Are all the objects we surround ourselves with on a daily basis necessary for life, or are they only objects that teach us how to be helpless? Is it not sometimes the case that we become victims of gadgets? Of course, I am not an extreme conservative, and I do not think that technical civilization and progress are the same evil. Of course, I am aware that the achievements of civilization save human life and health. Unrestricted access to knowledge makes humanity able to overcome the diseases that decimated whole nations centuries ago. But each stick has two ends. After all, it is also an undeniable fact that most of us, left alone without a mobile phone, without batteries for a flashlight, without breathing clothes or freeze-dried food in the middle of the forest, during hot summer or cold winter, would die of exhaustion after a few days. Most of us would not be able to get food or find shelter. We wouldn't be able to survive. Why wouldn't we be able to survive? Well, the objects around us made us dependent on their functionality and usefulness. Without them, we wouldn't be able to cope with the harsh conditions of harsh nature, which, of course, provides us with food and shelter if we can get them. But it also does not forgive mistakes. Surely you have heard of people who just died from the cold because they couldn't dry their clothes soaked during a downpour. However, death from a cold is only an effect and not a reason for not surviving in the deaf. The real reason is the mentality of modern man, who trusts too much in technology. Did you know that some people died because they got lost walking down a trampled path in the Oregon forest and because they couldn't help themselves to eat raw fish or a small rodent that they could easily hunt? When the supplies ran out, they stood helpless in the midst of the humming trees, falling into despair.

In 1989, Cyclone Hugo struck the southeastern coast of the United States and went further inland than any other cyclone in history. Many people lost their lives, and entire cities were razed to the ground. Many people who lived so far inland never imagined that a cyclone could have such an impact on them and put them in danger of life and health overnight.

Until then, they thought that only the coastal residents had anything to worry about. I was amazed at how many people seemed helpless. But there were also those who did not allow their minds to succumb to the paralyzing helplessness. Moreover, they helped each other, evoking a sense of community that had never been seen before. It took a tragedy like Cyclone Hugo to bring out the best in some people. Unfortunately, the worst was also when neighbors took advantage of the misfortune their community had suffered and plundered destroyed houses. Unfortunately, sometimes it takes a tragedy to reveal our true nature.

How about you? Are you a person who would survive a similar cataclysm or rather become its victim? Ask yourself, what would you do if you were to face danger? A truly determined survivor will continue to fight for survival at all costs. He'll certainly not take into account what he's lost or the anguish he's experiencing. He'll just leave what he's lost and find a way to deal with the new circumstances. It is this style of behavior that has actually helped people face the circumstances of the past and has given them the power not only to survive but also to rebuild the lifestyle they have lived in the past. Too many have neglected or never discovered what a true blessing it is to simply live. If you know how to deal with small troubles and can appreciate small pleasures, you'll live a better life, because you'll know that nothing really valuable comes easily. In a scenario of having to survive in new conditions, whether it be a natural disaster, a major economic crisis, a pandemic, or a war, taught by the experience gained in calmer times, you will also be able to cope with a critical situation.

The will to survive, a determination will be natural for you. Because I want to assure you that you can give more of yourself than you think, initially, learn to discover in yourself skills that you had no idea existed. While there is still time to test solutions that will help you when it comes to testing.

you must have at least 1 liter per person per day if your survival kit is to be easy to carry. A 1-gallon bottle would use too much space, leaving too little room for other essential products and would add an extra 25 pounds of weight to what you would have to carry. Since your survival kit should last you at least three days, you will need to have three 1-liter bottles of water in your bag. Also, remember to pack a few items to help you collect and filter the water. A foldable, compact bucket can help you to collect water from the jet or collect rainwater. To clean the water, you should boil it and, if you have one, you should use iodine tablets. Of course, if you have the right filters, you can clean the water even more. You should boil the water for at least 5 minutes, but it is better to boil it for 20 minutes. There are ways to boil water without a pot or kettle, but I suggest you buy a small jug with a lid. This will not only be useful for boiling water. You can use it to store smaller items or coffee, tea, or sugar.

Food

There are many kinds of high-energy foods - like energy bars - that you should get. Of course, make sure the food has a long shelf life, as long as you are obviously careful to avoid food poisoning. Pay attention to freeze-dried meals, as their volume is smaller than that of traditional meals, and their nutritional value is not less. To prepare such a meal you need only water. There is a wide range of such products on the market so everyone will find something for themselves. Do not forget to have a few dishes to prepare a meal. It is best made of plastic because it does not break and is lightweight. Just make sure that it is resistant to high temperatures and quite durable. It may happen that for a long time, you will not be able to replace such a plate or mug.

Clothes

You must have several types of clothes in your bag to protect yourself in case you fall into a river or get wet during a downpour. As I have already written above, it is not so hard to get a cold because of wetness, and it was stupid to come down from this world for such a trivial reason as the lack of trousers or a shirt for a change. You may have to walk many miles every day, so your rescue kit should include an extra pair of comfortable shoes. Best of all, those that you've been wearing so as not to surprise yourself or suffer from abrasions. .A few sets of woolen socks and long underwear will keep you warm for a long time. A few sets of woolen socks and long underwear will keep you warm for a long time. You don't have to have super-durable, professional trekking clothes with you. It would be something comfortable and durable, which will not tear on the first bushes you meet. Remember to pack 2-3 shirts with long sleeves. Remember that a long sleeve shirt can also function as a short sleeve shirt only by rolling up the sleeves. However, short-sleeved shirts will not change into long-sleeved shirts if it is necessary. I think a light raincoat might come in handy too because you certainly don't want to get wet. Especially when there's nowhere to dry soaked clothes.

Finally, don't forget your hat. No survival package is complete without a hat. You can opt for a Crocodile Dundee look, a woolen hat, or even a baseball hat that will protect you from the sun and keep some of your precious warmth from escaping from your head.

Shelter

You should have some durable, waterproofing material in your equivalent kit to cover your shelter if necessary. Make sure that this tarpaulin has reinforced air vents, that you can tighten the roof, and that it is made of polyester or nylon. A five-person tent with the extra room is unlikely to be practical. Alternatively, you might think of a small, foldable one-person tent with a sturdy cord and duck tape, which can be used in countless cases. If there is still some space in your bag, think about packing a thermal blanket or aluminum foil.

First-aid package

Several types of first aid packages can be purchased for emergency use. The basic first-aid kit will do the job. I recommend that you add a book on standard first aid to the first-aid package in case you have never received first aid training. Having all the patches, bandages, bands, descaling agents, without proper knowledge of how to use them, can end in an unpleasant surprise.

Everything else

You should adapt your survival kit to the situations in which you are most likely to find yourself, based on the topography of the terrain in which you will find yourself, with all the important places like rivers, hills, or points that can be used as a shelter if necessary. You cannot forget your survival knife made of high-quality steel so that it does not blunt too easily. You will need waterproof matches, a few lighters, and a flint stick, as well as a few flashlights. These can be battery-powered or small crank models, but if they are battery-powered, don't forget the extra batteries. A small sewing package with a durable sewing needle can be useful. A few flares will come in handy when you need to signal your whereabouts. Think of a fishing kit. Catching a fish when you're hungry can greatly increase your morale and even save lives. A compass is as useful as possible if you know how to use it. A multi-tool will certainly be useful, especially as it is unlikely to take up much space.

Just in case, pack a small amount of money. You just never know...

I've indicated the survival package above, which you can, of course, modify as you wish. Try to predict which scenarios are the most probable, and that's what to do when choosing your equipment. Even if you are not perfectly prepared - and something will certainly surprise you - you will still be much better prepared than most people.

How You Can Optimize Your Readiness To Survive

———

I believe that having a survival strategy developed is at least as important as packing all the necessary items into a prepared bag. A strategic plan is therefore crucial because even without a bag of useful items, you are able to survive during a disaster, as long as you have a previously developed strategic plan in case of a disaster or other critical event. In this chapter, I will focus on how to maximize our readiness for survival by analyzing how to conduct a strategic evacuation.

Before developing a strategy for survival, we need to analyze several elements:

1. What disasters can happen at your location?

An important component of survival preparedness is understanding what has happened in your area in the past. Is your location known for mass floods? Do you live in an area with earthquakes or mudslides? Has your city ever been the target of a terrorist attack? Think about these aspects when making a plan; they can immediately eliminate some choices or make others more beneficial.

2. What are your strengths and weaknesses?

Thinking about your strengths and weaknesses can help you adapt your survival strategy to what you are really good at and what you absolutely need to improve. This analysis of your characteristics will greatly increase your chances of survival. Is your physical fitness above average, or should you improve this aspect? If your overall fitness is high, you will be able to plan longer routes or more weight of the bag you take with you. Can you give first aid? It can be extremely important if the person you are traveling with has an accident and is seriously injured. Identifying your weaknesses can be just as important as understanding your survival skills. Can you light a fire in difficult conditions? Can you control your direction at night? Can you use a map and a compass? Do you know the fauna and flora in your area well? Learning all these things and realizing what else needs improving will make you really well prepared.

Remember that the more skills you have, the fewer things you need to have with you.

3. The location of your refuge in building your survival strategy plays a vital role. It will have a huge impact on your morale, your sense of security, and will give you the comfort of choosing different solutions depending on the situation. It is best to plan 4 locations, each one in a different direction from the perspective of where you are. If a catastrophe happens and it turns out that your shelter to the East of you has been destroyed, you always have three other directions (West, North, and South) where you can go. Will you ask what could be such a spare location? It could be your relative's house, your holiday home, the mall, the underground garage, or your son's or daughter's school. Look at the map and try to mark these places on it. You can also plan the location of your inventory in these places and along the roads leading to them so that you don't have to move everything you own from place to place every time. Besides, it gives you the comfort of knowing that if you lose some of your inventory, you always have more of them, located in different places. This is a kind of resource diversification strategy, according to the principle "don't put all the eggs in one basket," so important in business, for example.

4. Calculate how long it will take you to move from place to place.

Travel time is crucial for your safety. If you can determine your average speed, you will know how many days or hours it will take you to reach your destination, so you will know how many things you need to survive to eat, drink and sleep on the way. Your average speed will be most affected by the following variables:

Weight of your bag - An average person can bring no more than 25 to 30 percent of their body weight in a backpack. As you prepare, test your abilities and move the bag over a certain distance, packing enough things into it so that the weight of the bag corresponds to that of the day when something bad happens. You must be able to carry your bag for several hours, if not days. I don't think you need to carry out such an experiment to know that exceeding the bag's weight by far will make it impossible for you to get away efficiently when necessary.

Analyzing the terrain, you will be passing through - The average speed of movement of an adult, healthy person with a backpack of the weight I indicated above is 2.5-4 miles per hour. Of course, when moving on flat ground. When considering your route, you need to be aware of what kind of surface you will have under your feet. People usually make the mistake of thinking that hiking downhill is more comfortable than going uphill. This is generally not true, because hiking downhill with a backpack means that you need to be very careful to have the right posture and to descend on slightly bent knees in order not to overload your joints and cause an injury. If your route is crossed by a reservoir, take into account the fact that the pace of your movement will then drop significantly.

5. Your general physical condition - it is quite obvious that a healthy, fit person will travel longer in a given unit of time than a sick and unfit person. You have to be realistic and plan your travel time according to your abilities.

Improving your physical condition usually takes weeks or months, depending on your starting point. So don't hesitate and start training today.

If you are moving to a larger group, you should include helping the elderly and children in your plan. Then adjust the time and pace of movement to the least fit, slowest person.

Other factors you should consider:

Plan to pack additional, preferably laminated maps with marked destinations and place them on different people. In addition, it is useful to mark landmarks along each route to facilitate navigation.

If you want to meet other people at a given location, create a map of routes, leading from different starting points of the journey to one common place where everyone can meet. By doing this in advance, you will avoid wasting everyone's precious time desperately trying to make contact with each other while you should have been on your way.

In addition, write down all phone numbers for your friends, colleagues, and emergency calls, copy and forward them to all members of the group. There is a chance that even during a disaster, the mobile phone network will continue to work for some time.

Remember that when packing your bag, you will have to make a choice between the items, each of which is useful. But be realistic. Although an axe or other heavy tool will be 100% useful, you will have to leave it to carry a weapon, for example. Always consider the probability of using a particular tool and object; it will allow you to make a good choice. I've already written about the fact that we take things to the camping site with us, which makes us not only look idiotic but simply make our lives more difficult? A battery-powered tent fan? No, definitely leave it at home.

Remember to always reach the place where you will be staying 2-3 hours before sunset. This will give you enough time to find a dry place sheltered from the wind, where you can pitch your tent, prepare food and water, and light a fire.

If you carry an optimally packed backpack, know that a person who weighs 160 pounds consumes over 400 kilocalories of energy during 1 hour of trekking. This is an effort level that can be compared to jogging. Always take a break to replenish your fluids and relax.

Conclusion

Building a strategic plan for survival is a key element in preparing for natural disasters or nuclear power plant failures such as the one in Fukushima, Japan. Remember that the fewer things you leave to faith, the greater your chance of survival and that of your loved ones.

Physical Preparation

T rain your body for the possibility of carrying heavy loads and covering long distances. Proper physical training will increase your chances of survival and survival significantly.

Understanding what condition your body is in will make you really assess your abilities, without having to make an effort that is beyond your strength.

Having a slender, muscular and resilient body that is a solid base for your overall condition shouldn't just result from a vain, self-centered need to please others, but above all from the belief that whether you have to go 10 or 20 miles, you can still do it without special effort.

We are evolutionarily predisposed to cross our limits of physical fitness, which makes us the most dangerous predators on Earth. In a threatening situation, the notion of competition and natural selection also becomes particularly important. This is when the most efficient and healthy individuals have the best chances for survival.

If we do not allow ourselves to become lazy by subjecting ourselves to various amenities resulting from the progress of civilization and let our instincts speak, we will feel that we have to work on our physical strength and exceed our capabilities.

We are all certainly familiar with Charles Darwin's concept that, in the long term, only the strongest and best-adapted individuals will be able to survive in their natural environment. They will be able to improve their qualities and pass them on to future generations.

Looking at where man is today and seeing that he has basically completely dominated other species on Earth, the concept of natural selection is definitely covered in reality.

About 100,000 years ago, the man reached its evolutionary peak; mankind has developed all the tools necessary for survival in the natural environment.

Our bodies have reached a point of development where it has become clear that we can not only survive in a demanding environment but also develop further and change the environment according to our changing needs.

So at one point, when our bodies and intelligence reached their peak of development, we realized how to manage our environment.

Our bodies and the biological mechanisms that have allowed us to survive for thousands of years have remained virtually the same, so that today, as the environment changes under our influence, among other things, we are able to adapt quite easily to these changes.

Let us remember that there are still mechanisms within us that used to enable us to escape or fight effectively many times. And although today our natural environment does not present us with such dramatic challenges as it used to, man is still able to face challenges and fight for survival at all costs. It seems that it is man's greatest skill, developed through evolution, that is the ability to prepare for the worst.

We are the best, the happiest and the healthiest when we are in an environment that regularly challenges us, forcing our body to adapt in order to overcome obstacles in the future in the most optimal way.

Unfortunately, living in big cities, traveling by comfortable means of transport, having more food than we need, safe roof over our heads, we do not feel pressure to improve our physical condition, seeing neither direct threats from other species nor the need to fight for every bite of food. Although the technological revolution has pushed the need to fight for existence into the background, let us remember that biologically we are the same as our ancestors who walked the Earth several decades ago.

However, as our natural environment made less and fewer demands on us, because, for example, we no longer had to fight with other species for food, we had to start to challenge ourselves to strengthen our bodies. We started to need specially designed training plans for us because our everyday life does not challenge us enough to get better and better.

If we are serious about surviving a possible cataclysm, we should ruthlessly get up from the table, turn off Netflix and go out into nature. Something that used to be natural for humans, i.e., the independent search for food, no longer exists today for known reasons. That is why we should at least partially return to the lifestyle of hundreds of years ago, when we spent most of our time outdoors, trying to somehow cope with the powerful nature, involuntarily improving our skills.

Physical training in the past was not about following a plan, but about doing things as usual and achieving better and better results in ever-changing circumstances.

And the result of perfect physical preparation was not a small reward or admiration of girls when we walked on the beach, but the preservation of health and often life.

Adequate physical training, which ensures the survival of the strongest individual, can be described as Optimal Physical Training.

Optimal Physical Training is a training that allows you to strengthen your body and stand out in your natural surroundings, which in turn allows you to cope with the unpredictable and diverse difficulties of life. It is not only a method to look better in a T-shirt or bathing suit.

At a certain level of the subconscious, we know that being fit for the environment is something positive, and being mismatched puts us in a very unfavorable starting position.

We also instinctively feel that the visible features of a healthy body are also evidence of strength and fitness.

We are naturally attracted to people who have a healthy, proportionally developed body, without visible overweight. We instinctively feel that such a person is the best partner for us, ensuring that our offspring receive the best evolutionary qualities.

People who have actually developed the ability to move around in the environment. They have no addictions, eat simple but healthy food, and regularly face difficult challenges, have a slim but muscular build, look younger than their physically inactive peers, healthy teeth, shiny eyes.

Of course, it is not about developing an attractive appearance for him. At least from the point of view of qualities necessary for survival. Rather, it's about optimizing the resources to ensure our safety.

A good, attractive appearance should be a natural consequence of taking care of his physical condition because if it is an end in itself, we can easily go to aesthetic surgery and give up running 10-15 miles a day. It is simply a matter of our personal choice. So far, it is legal to improve your beauty with a plastic surgeon's scalpel. It's a different matter what consequences it may have for physical and mental health, but this is already a topic for another book.

It is interesting what changes take place in the body and mind of a person who regularly exercises.

Not only does the body function better, and the phenomenon of metabolic transformation takes place more efficiently, but also on the mental level, there are obviously beneficial changes. For example, in the area of social functioning, greater self-confidence, belief in one's skills, and less risk of affective disorders. Of course, it is not advisable to generalize, but you will admit that you do not need advanced medical knowledge to conclude that a slim, fit, smiling person is less exposed to the diseases of civilization than someone who eats only highly processed food and rarely moves from his couch.

The aim is to reverse the unfavorable changes that take place in your body, which result, among other things, from insufficient physical activity. After all, it is never too late in life to introduce beneficial changes. The reward will be not only a better physical and mental well-being, but also greater effectiveness in dealing with the adversities of fate when one day you wake up in a completely new, much more difficult and perhaps even horrifying reality.

How To Light A Fire

———

If you've ever been in a situation where you have to fight for survival, especially in humid or cold weather, a few things will be just as important to your survival as the absolutely crucial ability to light a fire. Remember the chapter where I wrote about hypothermia? Hypothermia can occur when your body temperature drops by only 2 degrees, and there is no need to mention that fire can be what stands between you and freezing to death. A big, hot fire can make a difference more than anything else in this situation. However, lighting a fire, especially if you don't have matches or a lighter, can be difficult at best. Mastering such a skill at a time of mental tension and when it is slowly getting dark will be practically impossible if you have never invested enough time in developing the skill of lighting a fire in difficult weather conditions.

So now it's time to present the methods of making a fire. Let my instructions serve as part of your ability to start a fire, and you will need to repeat the same actions many times. Remember that the weather is never the same and the weather conditions can change in a few minutes. Exercising this skill is all the more important because there will be no time to flick through the guides if you have to light a fire quickly. You need to master the skill at such a level that you don't think too much about what you are doing. Just as you don't analyze every move in depth while driving. It's just a matter of muscle memory, and sometimes it takes a lot of repetition to achieve this. You can't count on you to save yourself or someone else if you don't understand enough.

Where to light a fire?

Location is extremely important when it comes to where you cross the river, where you set up your camp, and the same goes for choosing where to light a fire. There are many things to think about:

Where do you want to build a hut or a tent? After all, the fire is not only to warm you up or prepare a meal but also to light up the place where you have decided to stay the night. If possible, pitch a tent under a pitched tree, where the lowest branches are at least 10 feet high. This will minimize the risk of sparks jumping from the fire to the branches and start a fire. This could happen, so try to estimate the risk as closely as possible.

Which side is the wind blowing from? You don't want the blast to set off a sheaf of sparks and direct them to your tent. Ideally, if this place is well covered, then there is a good chance that your fire will burn evenly and that the smoke won't make your life miserable.

What are the ground conditions? On the damp ground, the fire will have difficult conditions, if you manage to light it at all. In snowy or wet areas, you may need to create a base on which you can build a stable and dry fireplace. Build an elevation from the available stones, or build an earthwork to prevent water from melted snow and ice from putting out the fire.

Of course, protect the surrounding vegetation, trees, and bushes and yourself from the fire. Clean the place where you want to light a fire from all the dry vegetation that could get into the fire while you sleep. You'd better not be suddenly trapped in a fiery circle. Fist-sized stones form a perfect ring around the fire, use them.

You can't count on a decent bonfire without fuel. If you're just in a wooded area, you probably have plenty of dry branches that are perfect for starting a fire. However, the best thing to do is to have dried out trees that have not yet been blown over by the wind, as there is no risk of them being wet as the branches that absorb moisture from the ground can be. If you're not lucky enough to find a tree for firewood, remember that dried excrement from large animals is also suitable to fuel the fire. The North American Indians did just that when they had to light a fire in the open air, the prairie. They used dry buffalo droppings for this purpose. Or you can mingle dry rhizomes, grass. Tightly tangled, they would burn longer than if they were loose. Whatever you find, guess enough to keep the fire going. However, there is a risk that the fire will go out in the morning because you can't predict exactly how much wood you need.

A fire starter. Finding a dry fire starter in a damp autumn forest is quite a challenge. If you were to light a fire in your home fireplace, you could use paper as a fire starter. However, when camping, you have little chance of finding dry paper nearby. Finding the right material for the fireplace will be crucial when setting up the camp. Try to look for something in the area. Even a tree that has fallen over in wet bushes can hide material dry enough underneath to catch fire. Dry grass is also perfectly suitable for this. If there is no dry grass, twigs, or leaves nearby, take a knife and scrape off the log, from bottom to top, to form a spongy mulch from the deadwood. You can also use a knife to remove the bark from the first better branch, and this will get you into drier wood.

Your own clothes can also provide you with firewood.

Make a small ball of fabric fiber, then place a small pile of wood chips on top of it and try to set it on fire while protecting it from the wind. If you find a fallen furry animal or dry moss nearby, you can also use it as a firefighting material. Of course, you can also use it as a firewood material. It is perfect if there are some brushwood and thicker branches to fuel the fire.

You can also make sure you have a dry fire starter with you beforehand. It doesn't have to be anything special. You can buy a barbecue fire starter, or some kind of flammable liquid, at the first gas station.

You can use the following ideas for making the fire starter yourself:

- Cotton balls covered with Vaseline (put them in a plastic bag so as not to soil the rest of the stuff in your bag or backpack).

- Pieces of pine wood, covered with resin

- Clothes scraps - while still at home, find the unnecessary part of the peel, cut into pieces and place at the bottom of your survival bag, that's when they will prove very useful.

Use petroleum-based Vaseline or some kind of drug, like WD40, a two-component adhesive, epoxy resin, motor oil, cosmetics in the aerosol. Try to combine several ingredients. This will have a better effect than if you use each one separately. Add wood chips, pieces of bark, anything of organic origin to this mixture and make a ball out of it all. You'll be surprised how a homemade fire starter works. You can count on the fact that such a fire starter will burn longer, which will give you more time to start a bigger fire. In addition, the heat from such a fire starter can dry up a pile of wood, which you can place over it.

You are wondering how to start a fire at all if you don't have matches or a lighter with you.

I'm sure it's not the kind of problem you'd want to deal with if you're facing a life-threatening threat...

But, well, it could happen anyway. And I have good news for you. There are many ways to light a fire without matches.

But for now, get ready.

Gather the twigs in a bunch, just like you gather wildflowers. Keep the thicker ends together at the bottom; the narrower ends face up. Build a small pile to resemble an Indian tipi. Place a prepared fire starter inside it. Now you're ready to start creating the sparks from which the fire starter should light up.

If someone asked me what my first association with lighting a fire without matches is, it would be friction. The friction of one object against another increases the temperature between the rubbed objects and leads to ignition. Of course, as you can guess, these can't be any objects. Rubbing plastic cutlery against each other is unlikely to cause the flames to light up after a while in the dark.

The easiest way to cause a fire is to rub a piece of flint against high carbon steel. There is a good chance that your knife is made of this steel. To find the flint go down the stream, as long as it flows nearby. With a bit of luck, you should find pieces of flint.

Another method is to start a fire using a lens that focuses the sun's rays. I'll tell you right away that this method will definitely not work if you want to focus on the flammable material, moonlight, or starlight.

Generally, this technique is quite simple. Many little boys have mastered it to perfection by torturing ants that were unreasonable enough to wander in their vicinity with sunlight concentrated in the lens. The biggest disadvantage of this method, as I mentioned, is that you need a sunny day to use it.

Okay, but how am I supposed to tie a lens?

Maybe you took your binoculars, camera, flashlight, or glasses with you. Yeah, you can use the lenses taken out of these things to light a fire. It may not be possible to restore these objects to their original state, but in a life-threatening situation, such dilemmas come to the fore.

Hold the lens in such a way and at such an angle that the sunlight passing through it concentrates in the form of a small, bright point on the arson. You can also try not to destroy your binoculars by pointing the wider end to the sun and the narrow end to something you want to set fire to. You should be able to see how you have to hold the lens, and with a bit of patience, you should see the smoke after a while, which shows that you were holding your hand still.

It is very important to take a fixed position because the whole idea is to focus the narrow beam on something flammable for a few dozen seconds.

This may seem ridiculous to you, but in extreme cases, even ice can be used as a lens.

So you can use a piece of ice, which is clean and transparent. Use a knife to form a 2-inch piece of ice into a lens. You can also use a stone to grind a piece of ice and give it the desired shape. The temperature of your fingers will probably be higher than the temperature of the ice, so gently smooth the edges of the ice, leaving the center a little thicker. Then use the prepared piece to focus the sunlight exactly as you did with a conventional lens.

Another way to focus the sunlight is to use a piece of aluminum to make a can of your favorite drink. You have to make the piece of aluminum to be polished to a high gloss. This is not particularly difficult. Use fine sand, toothpaste, or even chocolate to polish the aluminum. A mirror prepared in this way, set at the right angle, will reflect the sun's rays, and there is a good chance that a small smoke will appear after a while.

Another method is to use a bottle with clean water. The bottle can also turn into a lens, as long as it holds it is facing the sun and the firelight, at the right angle, of course. Don't forget to remove the label. The surface of the bottle must be perfectly transparent.

If you have a transparent plastic bag with you, fill it with clean water to create a bulging shape. As you can guess, this will give you a lens-like surface. Continue with the examples I gave you earlier.

TIP: Focusing the light beam on a darker surface is much more effective than on a bright one. If you don't have anything dark and are wearing a darker shirt or, for example, a black glasses cleaning cloth, you can use the fragment to focus the sunlight.

Remember, you have to be creative. As you see for yourself, there are many solutions that are not obvious. Just take a look around and test a few solutions; something will finally work. Don't give up.

How to light a fire. - Other methods

If you carry a battery and a piece of aluminum foil or wire, you can also light a fire if you don't have a match or a lighter. This is one of the simplest alternative methods of lighting a fire. Even a battery as small as AA will work. Make a longer piece of aluminum foil or wire so that both ends touch the poles of the battery. The resulting combination will make the wire expand almost instantly, igniting the previously prepared fire starter. You can use aluminum from the chewing gum package but be prepared for the fact that such a piece of aluminum is quite thin and delicate and therefore burns out very quickly.

In any of these methods - and I'm sure we haven't exhausted the subject - it's very important to catch the moment when a small flame is created. Try not to suppress it, especially since you've gone to great lengths to bring it about. Blow gently, add sticks, pieces of wood, dry grass, then branches and thicker logs.

Congratulations! You made a fire!

I have a piece of advice for you - practice firing the fire as often as you can. Just training makes the master. That way, when you really need a fire, you'll do it without hesitation.

If your son, daughter, colleague, anyone is with you, do it together. For it's a good thing if more than one person we might have to run away with at some point has been able to light a fire.

Good luck!

How To Prepare Light And Cheap Meal

To be in good shape, a person must have not only a varied diet, but also an adequate amount of it. The food, especially the food we want to pack in an escape rucksack or one for a short trip, can be heavy. And yet we know perfectly well that moving with a load is an additional energy expense, as well as less space in your luggage. So what can be done to minimize not only the weight but also the volume of the food being carried? The easiest solution will be:

- reduce the amount of water in the food products,

- reduce the weight of the packaging.

Military rations, although they are nutritious, are not cheap or generally light. Unless you decide to take only selected products with you. They also contain a lot of preservatives to extend their shelf life. You can also reach for freeze-dried sets. Thanks to this method, products are effectively protected against spoilage, while maintaining their nutritional values to a significant extent. Freeze-dried products are lighter and take up less space than their conventional counterparts. They are packed as single or double portions. Their preparation is quick: just pour hot or hot water over them and wait a while. Unfortunately, when buying several sets in detail, you have to reckon with a large expense.

In this case, one of the options will be to prepare the ingredients for meals by yourself. The cheapest solution is a mixture of cereals, i.e., self-made muesli. Ingredients are easily available in every grocery store:

- rye, wheat, oat, barley, corn,

- wheat bran,

- young barley (powder),

- dried fruit (e.g., sultanas, dates, apple, apricot, plum, forest fruit),

- milk powder,

- cocoa powder,

- sunflower seeds, and crushed nuts,

- cumin, expanded amaranth or expanded buckwheat.

This type of whole-grain muesli is a full-calorie meal, complete in every respect. You don't have to boil it, just pour hot water, stir it, and enjoy the valuable food. The lunch version can consist of several types of peas, pasta, instant buckwheat flakes, powdered root, matzo, and dried vegetables with spices. As an addition or snack (not for vegetarians!), it is worth taking jerky, i.e., dried meat, with you.

Tip! You can make dried jerky meat yourself. First, the meat (e.g., beef, turkey, horsemeat) should be thoroughly cleaned of fat, cut into thin longitudinal slices, and then dried a few hours above the heat and smoke to prevent it from spoiling. Usually, drying also involves adding salt and chili peppers to prevent the growth of bacteria in the meat.

Most bulk products can be poured into plastic bags (e.g., string bags), setting the appropriate portions. This will make it easier for us to plan sets for a prede-termined time.

Tip! You can pour some of the ingredients into an empty PET bottle. This will give you not only a stronger package but also an emergency water container.

It's really hard to live without electricity these days because practically every-thing requires electricity from a socket or a battery. A fridge, like many other appliances, is also dependent on a constant supply of electricity. Let's look at the solutions that will help you to keep your food products in the fridge for as long as possible. If you're planning on switching off the power supply for a longer period of time, for example, before you go to work, set your cooling to a low-er temperature than usual. This will store a cold reserve, increasing the cooling process for items already stored. And here's a curiosity: the more products are in the fridge and freezer, the longer they stay cold. So, if you have the possibility throw a few things into the free compartments of the freezer (they don't nec-essarily have to be food products). In particular, I recommend putting filled ice bags or PET bottles filled in three quarters with slightly salty water. Remember to keep the containers tight and tight. They will then act as cooling inserts and allow you to keep your food cool for longer. When you find that a refrigerator has no power supply and is unlikely to recover quickly, make a quick overview of what products should be consumed or thrown away right away, as they will start to spoil first. The shorter the fridge or freezer is opened, the less cold it will be lost. Be careful not to let warm air in from outside. The fridge or freezer then works like a thermos.

Interesting! Did you know that some manufacturers equip modern refrigerators with a temperature maintenance function? It is very useful in case of a power failure. Depending on the model, this parameter varies from several to several hours.

Until agriculture was established, all people on Earth fed on wild plants and animals. Their food was regional, organic, and seasonal. Currently, practically all city dwellers are dependent on food supplies from outside. Food products are available in shops and food wholesalers, as well as served as meals in bars and restaurants. But if one day all these establishments were closed, would you know where to get plant-based food from? In general, trees, shrubs, and other plants bear abundant fruit, and a large proportion of them can be used as food. It is best to use species that are known and proven. And there is no shortage of such species, especially in allotment gardens. Sometimes in parks or along roads, you can find fruit trees, as well as common or woody hazelnut, which will offer us hazelnuts in September and October.

Attention! Avoid eating fruit growing along roads with heavy traffic or near industrial plants, as many harmful pollutants have certainly penetrated them.

Interesting! Did you know that hazelnuts are a valuable product in terms of nutrition? They are rich in unsaturated fats, protein, and carbohydrates, so they are healthy and easily digestible food. Roasted hazelnuts can be stored for a very long time and under all conditions.

In difficult times we will probably have to eat also unconventional things, that is, things that our ancestors reached for, but which the generation brought up in the age of globalization no longer knows.

Acorns from common beech - this tree is very popular in many areas, it is also found in urban and suburban parks. Its fruit is a small walnut (beech) wrapped in a bowl covered with soft hair. When it ripens, the cover breaks into four parts, and the fruit falls out of it. This usually takes place from the end of August to October. Unfortunately, they are not among the tastiest - they are very sour. However, beechnuts are rich in assimilable iron, potassium, magnesium, and calcium. They have a lot of fat and just as much protein and some fiber in their composition. Slightly roasted beeches can be eaten directly, while strongly roasted and powdered, they are a substitute for coffee.

Acorns from oak - a tree equally popular. Its autumn fruits are rich in carbohydrates (starch), protein, and B vitamins. They also contain a lot of zinc and other macros- and microelements. Acorn flour can be used to bake bread or scones, roasted ones can be eaten on their own, and after being roasted and brewed, they successfully replace coffee. This one, known as acorn flour, does not contain caffeine or other alkaloids, but has a strengthening effect, causes a feeling of satiety, strengthens the stomach, spleen, and liver and generally regulates the digestive system. The fruit inside the shell is characterized by a strong bitter taste of tannin, which in larger quantities can harm us. To get rid of it, one should crush the testicle and rinse it in running water (river, brook) for the best 24 hours. In the case of limited water resources, the process of rinsing peeled acorns can be replaced by daily leaching in a solution of ash from deciduous trees.

At home, this can be done faster by boiling them in a weak ash solution and changing the water several times. Bitter tannins dissolve in water without any problem, and the more crushed acorns, the faster the process is. Put tannins-free acorns into a pot with water and boil. Then crush them and dry them, spread in a thin layer near a radiator or on a tray in an oven. Dried acorns can be ground into groats or fine flour. Such flour is best combined with another one (rye, wheat) so that not only one spicy taste dominates.

Tip! Oak acorns collected from the ground often contain larvae. These types of nuclei are no longer suitable for further processing, although the released worm can be used as bait for fish.

Pine cones - young, still green cones can be eaten as long as they are soft - it is best to boil or strangle them. Warm the mature cones to release seeds from them. They are tasty raw, but it is even better to roast them. From freshly obtained needles or young twig tips, you will get a vitamin C rich infusion.

Tip! You can prepare jam from young shoots and young pine cones. Mix the young green twig tips and cones in a blender or chop finely. Then cook over low heat in a small amount of sweetened (sugar or honey) water, stirring for about 15-20 minutes. Pour the resulting mixture into clean jars.

Maple seeds - seeds of common maple and sycamore are also edible. After peeling, they can practically be eaten raw, but it is recommended to roast or boil them beforehand. It is a popular park and estate tree. Due to its characteristic appearance, the leaves are easily recognizable.

Birch - the inflorescences and young leaves are suitable for eating, as they have diuretic, detoxifying, and metabolism-enhancing properties. The pulp and sap under the bark can be chewed raw, boiled or dried, powdered and added to flour or replaced. They are sweetest in spring, but can also be obtained later.

Interesting! Did you know that edible goat's mushrooms often grow near birch roots?

Nettle leaves - young nettles are collected before they bloom. Boil the young plant shoots for a few minutes to neutralize the formic acid in the hairs. In the past, nettles used to cook soup. The leaves are a source of vitamins, mainly A, C, and K (anti-hemorrhagic effect). They also contain mineral salts, among them as valuable as iron, potassium, silicon, and calcium. The leaves can be dried out and stored for a long time. The roots are rich in organic acids, phytosterols, lecithin, lignans, mucilages, and mineral salts.

Wateringerball - has long, narrow leaves and impressive dark brown flower shoots. It grows in ponds and lakes and on their banks. The rhizome and stems can be eaten raw, baked in ash, or boiled (boil the leaves like spinach and the young stems like asparagus). Pollen can be mixed with water for dough and baked or boiled. Even when the plants are already dried out, we are able to get the edible parts.

Did you know that baton down is also a good material for warming clothes as a filler? Because it's flammable, it's suitable as a kindling material.

Popular forest and field fruits are blueberry (including blackberry), elderberry, blackberry, hawthorn, rowanberry, wild rose, sea buckthorn, American cherry, raspberry, cranberry, and strawberry. Most of them are suitable for direct consumption or after short processing. Forest edible fruits are usually a low-calorie food but contain mineral salts and vitamins. The exception is hazelnuts, which have a higher percentage of protein than hen's egg.

Attention! Fresh rowanberries are bitter and tart and can cause vomiting and diarrhea. Therefore, they should first be thoroughly dried, boiled, or soaked for 24 hours in salted water before consumption. Another solution is to wait for frosts before the fruit is picked. However, if you have an efficient fridge, put the fruit in the freezer for the whole day - this will make it bitter.

Besides edible plants, there are also poisonous plants. You need to be able to distinguish between them. So it's better to stay hungry than to risk serious poisoning.

Survival is violence. It requires the flow of blood, the suffering of the victim, and the perseverance and cunning of the hunter. During natural disasters and warfare, when hunger looked into their eyes, people quickly changed their culinary tastes. Those who wanted to survive had to overcome their resistances and eat even their recent pets. Also, during the occupation or siege, pigeons, cats, rabbits, and dogs disappeared from the city streets. During the II World War, the phenomenon intensified - peaople ate fallen cows and horses. Mice and rats were also caught. Every piece of meat that made up a meal was valuable no matter what animal it came from.

At present, there are few "breeding" animals in the cities:

- cats,

- dogs,

- rodents (mice, rats, moles, minnows, hedgehogs),

- birds (pigeons, wild ducks, swans, ravens, crows),

- wild animals (in gardens and pet shops),

- horses, ponies (in stud farms).

In an emergency, you will probably have to hunt animals to save your family from starvation. However, you should choose those species that require the least amount of energy to catch. If you burn more calories than the hunted prey provides, you make a risky decision. The environment you are in will dictate what you should follow.

Most animals living in the city are not afraid of people, also because they feed them, often unknowingly throwing food away. With a strong sling, mousetrap, and/or net, you will be able to hunt down or catch animals in town. Most of this equipment can be bought in shops or prepared from materials collected at home, in storage, or in a basement.

Attention! Rodents and birds living in cities often carry dangerous diseases, so when you kill them, you need to make sure there are no signs of disease on their bodies. If there are no such traces, you should carefully bury the killed animal over the fire before cooking.

The principle of most traps is simple - they have the smell of bait to encourage the animal and then trap it or cause its death. Spring-loaded traps, available in supermarkets, are very effective, provided that they are positioned perpendicularly to the wall, and the bait is between the spring and the wall. Their advantage is that a dead animal (e.g., a rat) is not able to inform the members of its herd about the danger. Mice do not have neophobia like rats - over fear, they are overwhelmed by the unrestrained curiosity to look into every hole, so it is easier to catch them.

The Sherman-type elementary trap, used to catch small rodents, is a rectangular construction, into which food is poured and which closes when the rodent enters. Its advantage is its foldable structure and low weight.

Another way of catching a mouse is a movable footbridge with bait at the end, attached to a plastic bucket (e.g., with water). There is a path to it (e.g., a wide slat). Since the beginning of the footbridge is in front of the edge of the bucket and the mouse has easy access to it to reach the bait, it has to walk on a rocking slipway, and under its weight, it tilts, dropping the mouse into the bucket.

All types of traps should be discreetly inspected every few hours - a rodent or a bird trapped in the trap should be immediately killed in a humane way, not causing it unnecessary suffering. Wild animals have a small amount of fat in their body, so their meat becomes dry during roasting and is a poorer source of energy than meat of livestock. Compared to fats or carbohydrates, the most energy is consumed by protein digestion. Up to 30 percent of the energy obtained from proteins will be used to "convert" proteins into a form of energy use to the body - glucose.

What and how to fish effectively?

Fish meat is tasty and healthy because it contains proteins, fats, and vitamins, which is all we need for proper nutrition. There are known cases when castaways have been feeding only this way for weeks. Also, in our lakes, ponds, and rivers, there are still fish that you can try to catch. However, fishing is never an easy task - in general, apart from a good lure, it requires a lot of patience, which can be confirmed by anyone who has angled at least once.

If an emergency situation forces you to fish, you will certainly not have an advanced fishing kit. If you are lucky, you will find several hooks and a coil of line in your survival can. However, if your set does not include such items, you can make them out of what you have with you:

- You can make a temporary hook from a clip or hairpin, and for larger fish, from a pin from the opening mechanism of the aluminum can.

- Make the line from the paracord core.

- The float that holds the lure at a certain depth is made from the bark of a tree or a plastic element that does not sink. Sometimes you can just find it in the reeds.

In spring, you can expect fish closer to noon, as well as just afterward. In summer, a much better time to fish is dawn and dusk. Use an earthworm or an insect as a universal lure with a hook. In some places, a more effective way to get fish is to use a trap or net. This trap is very easy to make, just have any PET bottle after drink. Cut the bottle at the top, where it begins to narrow. Depending on the size of the fish we hunt, you can cut off a place with a thread, and cut the edges slightly with a knife, creating something like a little "sun." Then turn the severed neck to form a funnel. Put it into the rest of the bottle and fix it at the top. For this purpose, we use tape, clips, or staple it with a wire at least in two places. You can also cut out small teeth, which bent to prevent the funnel from falling into the bottom of the bottle. It is also worth thinking about immobilizing the submerged bottle somehow (e.g., with tape and string). To set a trap, pour some bread, flakes, or insects into it - something that will attract fish. It is best to set the trap in a place where they often swim.

The principle of operation is simple: it is easy for the fish to swim inside, but it is difficult to swim back out. A net, if you have one, will work well mainly in medium stream rivers and streams. Additionally, to use it, you need weights and floating buoys or a line hanging between the edges. Interestingly, some window curtains have a mesh structure very similar to fishing nets, so you can try using it as a replacement.

Tip! With a curtain made from an abandoned house and a strong line and stick, you can make a jiggle in a few minutes to catch a small fish.

This is an effective method of fishing, although often, in addition to the fish themselves, the net will get tangled up with branches and rubbish that can damage the mesh structure. Remember to take your net with you when you leave the campsite permanently so that animals and other people do not fall into it.

All freshwater fish are edible but must be cooked or baked. This will harm bacteria, viruses, and parasites that may be present in the fish.

Although each one of us has a different vision of hunting, especially in a survival situation, chasing after large animals will not always be possible or safe. Then, like more than 75 percent of people in the world, you will have to reach for insects (e.g., crickets, larvae, or ants) to supplement your diet with a nutritious snack. What is normal in Asia, most Americans still associate with something disgusting. According to specialists, the reason for this is in our cultural and social upbringing.

Did you know that scientists claim that everyone unconsciously eats more than half a kilo of insects a year anyway? Their trace amounts are found in many food products.

Specialists convince that it is worth reaching for them because they are easily digestible and have high nutritional values. Most of them are a source of protein, carbohydrates, fats, vitamins, and minerals. Insects are particularly rich in phosphorus, potassium, iron, copper, zinc, manganese, sodium, B vitamins and niacin. In turn, their chitin carapace is a polysaccharide, which acts on the human digestive system practically like fiber, supporting its work.

Did you know that the nutritional content of protein in crickets is up to 65 percent? In comparison, there are 22 percent chicken breasts and 19 percent protein in 100 grams of turkey meat.

Almost two thousand insect species and molluscs are considered edible.

- earthworms (before preparation, throw them in clean water for 20 minutes),

- grasshoppers,

- larvae (rich in protein; look for them under the bark of decayed trees),

- ants (edible at any stage of development),

- wasps (very dangerous to obtain; remove the sting before eating),

- grasshoppers,

- leeches,

- bees (edible at every stage of development; remove the sting before eating; you will also find honey in their nest),

- peregrine locusts,

- a vineyard snail (before preparing it, starve it for two days),

- field crickets (rich in calcium),

- dragonflies.

Do not eat insects that are bright (especially red) or too hairy - it is most likely a poisonous species. Although some insects can be eaten raw, it is advisable to heat them up first by boiling, frying, or baking them over the heat of the fire.

It's one thing to get the game or the plant you're eating, and making it fit to eat while retaining as much nutritional value as possible, is another. As long as

In the case of fruit and vegetables, eating them raw is advisable, while in the case of meat, more time and energy should be devoted to its preparation. Of course, in extreme situations, meat from animals, especially fish, can be eaten raw. However, due to the risk of pathogenic viruses and bacteria, as well as issues of assimilability, all specialists suggest that animal products should be heat-treated during baking, cooking, frying, grilling, or cooking. It also results in the temporary preservation of meat products.

Baking/grilling overheat - probably the easiest method to do, as all you need is a bonfire and the tool you hope for, or which will keep the meat on fire. Unfortunately, during this process, the fat is melted, and the meat of small animals becomes dry very quickly and thus less tasty. Roasting over a bonfire also has the disadvantage that it is easy to burn the meat. Infield conditions, the heating of the product is uneven - the outer layers heat up faster than the inner layers. If you have this possibility, use aluminum foil or tied green leaves to keep the juice inside the product. Place the food prepared in the heat of the fire.

Cooking in water - increases digestibility and consumption value and kills microorganisms. During this process, some valuable nutrients penetrate into the water, so instead of pouring it out, it is better to drink it. The longer it takes to cook, the more nutrients are lost in the food. It is therefore recommended to put the products into the boiling water immediately. However, when cooking broth, the meat should be placed in cold water. You can cook in almost any pot - even an aluminum can with a cut off the top will do the job in a survival situation. For more information about extreme water boiling, see the section on water.

Steam cooking - place the food on a perforated inset or in a basket hung over boiling water, under a cover, for a short time. This method will work well with most food products. When steaming, the temperature can reach up to 248 degrees F so the food boils quickly. Remember to cut meat or fish into small pieces before cooking. Steam dishes maintain higher levels of nutrients, vitamins, and minerals. They remain juicy, as there is minimal juice leakage from the product.

How to store food in the field?

It is fully feasible to store food safely away from the refrigerator or kitchen cupboard. The essence is to protect food products from insects, rodents, larger mammals, and the influence of weather conditions. Here are some useful tips:

- When you put your supplies in a bag, flies, ants, and other insects will not get into it. A foil net or a raincoat can be used as a bag, in which you can put a dish of food. Tighten the bag with string and hang it on a branch in the shade.

- A hole in the ground or a mountain stream may be used as a temporary refrigerator, but remember to attach the package.

- Open canned food, especially meat, should be eaten immediately.

- Dried meat (jerky) can be stored for a very long time in difficult conditions without losing its high nutritional value.

The setting of the jerky should take place outside the camp. Raw meat must be heat treated as soon as possible unless the ambient temperature is negative or close to zero.

What if all grocery stores were closed? If there is a natural disaster, a collapse of the economy, or the outbreak of war, the supply infrastructure is either out of operation or severely restricted. The resources of grocery stores are sold out or stolen by panicked people in the first days. So, where can you find alternative places where you can get food and drink?

- Spice shops (spices, herbs, canned fruit, nuts, sweets),

- tourist shops (freeze-dried meals, energy bars),

- sports and nutrition shops (energy bars, food supplements, fruit mousses, drinks),

- pet shops (seeds, animal feed, animals),

- gardening and agricultural shops (fruit bush seedlings, Vegetable seeds or sprouts),

- Liquor stores (alcohol, sweets),

- Veterinary practices (pet food),

- Fitness clubs (energy bars, food supplements, nutrition, drinks),

- Cinemas and theatres (sweets, corn grains, drinks)

- Drugstores (sweets, drinks),

- Pharmacies (medicines, food supplements, juices),

- Petrol stations (candy, drinks),

- kiosks (sweets, drinks),

- post offices (confectionery),

- building markets (drinks and vending machines),

- schools and universities (vending machines with sweets or drinks).

The longer the crisis lasts, the more basic products gain in value, and the value of money decreases. A good to meet the requirements of a fungible good has to be an object that is difficult to access (scarcity of occurrence) and thus reaches a high value per unit. If you have gas to charge your lighters, collect empty lighters - you will be able to exchange them for other needed products. Alcohol, cigarettes, coffee, children's milk, toilet paper, and medical knowledge have always been and will always be a valuable commodity in barter exchange. You can add batteries and chargers to this list.

Of course, there will also be those who will find quite good food in the trashcans standing right next to supermarkets or bazaars. It is worth looking into these places unless someone else is not able to breakthrough. Every day huge amounts of products are thrown there.

Remember that producing food on your own, to a limited extent, is also possible for city dwellers. In addition to herbs and sprouts, you can start growing potatoes without any problems with the land you have accumulated and access to water. Although they contain few calories, they have plenty of vitamins (especially vitamin C and beta-carotene), minerals, fiber, and protein. By eating them, we replenish almost all mineral deficiencies in our bodies. Your terrace, balcony, and even the flat roof of your house will be a suitable place to grow. Use every bit of your home to plant plants that will give you energy or even vitamins. If you have the opportunity, try to get a live goat that can eat and digest almost anything and is the perfect farm animal for tough times. The same goes for hens. Cultivating and keeping animals will help you survive, especially if you don't have supplies or anything to exchange.

If you're careful, consider buying your own, even a small plot of land, and growing various plants, including unusual ones like Jerusalem artichoke (tuberous sunflower). Since a potential looter usually steals only what he knows, he will not consider ornamental plants as edible.

How to extend the shelf life of food products

According to the Belgian Federal Food Safety Agency, products such as flour, pasta, white rice, hard yellow cheeses, coffee, and tea are fit for consumption even one year after the expiry date. The same is true for other products - some of them can be safely consumed a few days, weeks, or months after the expiry date indicated on the packaging.

Mould, unpleasant smell, or the presence of insects disqualify any food regardless of the expiry date.

Natural factors that cause permanent deterioration of food products, up to and including spoilage, or have an adverse effect indirectly are air, light, temperature, humidity, time-lapse, and microorganisms. However, there are proven ways of prolonging the shelf-life without major deterioration in the nutritional value of the product: - Keep products in tight containers, in a dry, cool, and dark place. The higher the temperature or humidity, the shorter the shelf life.

- Store grain in its shells in an appropriate manner - it must "breathe." The room and container in which the grain is stored must be well ventilated. The grain must not be kept in plastic bags and containers that are airtight.

- Choose the freshest products for storage from this year's harvest.

The purpose of food drying is to reduce the water content of food so that enzymatic and life processes of microorganisms cannot take place, and therefore bacteria that cause food spoilage cannot develop. The advantage of the method is the simple preparation of such products, their low weight for easy transport and long shelf life.

Freezing consists of rapid cooling of the food product to a negative temperature and maintaining it during the entire storage period. It stops the development and action of microorganisms, also slows down the course of chemical reactions and enzymatic and biochemical processes. The advantage of this method is the appearance of the food after thawing and preservation of more vitamins and minerals than with traditional hot air drying. No salt or sugar needs to be added. An obvious disadvantage is a need for constant access to the cooling device.

Curing is the process of preserving meat using paleosols, a mixture of salt and sodium nitrite. Cured meat is used as intended, i.e., it is smoked.

We can also preserve food products by sugar concentration. The addition of sugar to food effectively inhibits the development of most bacteria and, with a large amount of it, even the development of mold. With home-made fruit, we make jams and jams by cooking and thickening. Pickling is an old and proven method of food preservation, which is based on the fermentation process, which takes place under the influence of bacteria that break down sugars into lactic acid and inhibits, among other things, the rotting process. The most important is salt, which accelerates lactic fermentation. Of course, cucumbers and cabbage (white, red, Italian) are best suited for ensiling, although asparagus beans, courgettes, and beets can also be successfully ensiled.

Spices - seasoned with sweet peppers or chili and pepper, the meat is able to stay fresh twice as long even without refrigerator. This is because these spices contain so-called antioxidants (antioxidants), which delay the spoilage of meat during the oxidation process.

Tip! Wrap raw meat in nettle leaves, which are then wrapped in parchment paper and placed in a cool place. This way of preservation allows the meat to be stored for 1-2 days. The formic acid contained in the nettle leaves has a preservative effect.

Did you know that if you prepare your food properly and provide them with optimal conditions, their usefulness can be significantly extended compared to what the regulations or the producer suggest on the packaging?

How to open a can without an opener?

I guess there is nothing more annoying for a hungry person than finding a canned food and not being able to open it. Fortunately, some multi-purpose penknives have a kind of opener. In general, however, the probability of getting a can opener under certain conditions may be less than finding another unopened can. In such a situation, you have to improvise effectively. If you are sure of the blade strength of your knife, use this tool. If you do not have any blade with you, try the following method:

- Find a strong, flat, and rough surface (e.g., pavement slab, concrete wall, or flat stone).

- Grasp the tin can by the bottom, and with the tip side three times as much as possible against the surface to wipe off the jointing point of the cover.

- Within a few minutes of intense friction, the lid should only hold on small pieces. Now it is enough to undermine it slightly.

Do not try to heat tightly closed canned food, as this can lead to uncontrollable bursting and burning with hot content from people sitting close to the fire.

Another method is to use even a blunt tool (e.g., a spoon) and make a moving motion around the inner shell with great pressure. As time goes by, the metal of the can should recede.

The military can openers are available - despite their low price and small size, they are effective, and their use will protect your knife from blunt. Interestingly, since 1942 they have been worn by U.S. Army soldiers on chains of immortals or keys and are also part of survival kits. A Swedish version is also available - heavier but more solid than the American prototype. Perfect as a key ring or pendant, it will fit into any wallet - it is always worth having one with you.

When your body feels that it is running out of supplies and you are delaying the delivery of food to it, your brain sends you a reminder to force you to eat. Hunger in the first days is largely a state of mind. There are a few tricks that will help you to silence the bubbling hunger for a while:

Chewing gum - by chewing food (in this case gum), even if you don't swallow it, you send a signal to your brain to reduce your appetite. Chewing for too long, stimulates the secretion of gastric acids and thus causes a feeling of hunger.

Drink something warm - cold or lukewarm water will not help as well as warm. It can be green or black tea, which you can even sweeter, especially if you know that your glucose level has dropped sharply. Herbal infusions fight hunger perfectly. I especially recommend mint or lemon balm - not only do they force the body to forget about the recent desire to snack something, but they also raise our immunity. Water fills the stomach, giving a feeling of satiety for a short time. However, do not drink salted water, excess salt damages the kidneys!

If you have some food, eat smaller portions, enjoying every bite and chewing carefully. This will overcome hunger very effectively.

Avoid salty food - salty food increases your appetite.

Did you know that citrus aroma, especially grapefruit and lemon, blocks the receptors responsible for the feeling of hunger in our brain? The scents of conifers will work in a similar way.

At the initial stage of your diet, you will probably still be hungry and weakened. But if this period lasts longer, in 3-4 days, your body will adapt to the changes. Undernourishment lasting more than 14 days leads to a decrease of 20 percent in the basic metabolic rate because shrinking stocks are not able to meet the needs of the body.

The Misconceptions That Are Your Worst Enemy.

Having a survival kit alone will not guarantee your survival. Once you understand this, the probability of making glaring mistakes will be much less. Good preparation will also result in fewer negative surprises. With this in mind, you will put more effort into improving your skills.

Here are eight myths about the rescue kit that you can believe:

1. I will always have a rescue kit with me.

This is not proof of realism. Imagine, for example, that you are at work, and your rescue kit is at home. There is an earthquake, the highways are blocked, people are panicking around, and you are standing helpless and angry at yourself that you only have empty drink cans in your car. You thought you were prepared, you collected all the necessary equipment and left it at home. Unfortunately, you won't be able to use it anymore, especially since your house might have ceased to exist.

Your plan

Throw a smaller bag in the car. There's probably not everything in it that's in your primary bag left at home. But it's better than nothing. Let it be some little back with a first aid kit, a flashlight, a little money, a map of the area, a bottle of water. Throw that backpack in the trunk. I hope you never have to use it.

2. My rescue package will help me survive any disaster.

And what if the disaster lasts seven days? It's great to have a rescue package. But how long can your rescue kit last? One day? Three days? Four days? How about just a few hours? How do you even know how long it'll all take?

Your plan

Plan for the next 72 hours after the crash and prepare boxes in different places where you can hide your most important things. This will allow you to have access to food, water, batteries, etc. when the first three days after the crash have passed. The idea is to pack something lightweight in a handbag that will allow you to survive the first hours. You should plan to store your supplies in places that are reasonably easy for you to access, which may be difficult. Of course, you'll do all this under the assumption that you can't get home.

3. The contents of my rescue kit will help me survive any disaster.

The problem is that something may come up that will totally surprise you. In 2020, this thing is a coronavirus pandemic. Had you have expected something like this six months ago? The problem is that many of the ready-made sets that you can buy online include very basic equipment. Let me give you an example. One day I was watching Ebola survival kits on a website. I came across them by accident; I didn't even know that someone was offering something like this. What does a sample survival kit contain? A one-person folding tent, a few pairs of rubber gloves, and a survival whistle. I can assure you that it wouldn't save anyone in the event of ANY epidemic. And you see, the equipment that was supposed to save your life, and it costs a lot, is totally useless.

Your plan

Don't rely on a set that someone else has put together. If you anticipate a particular type of disaster in your location, prepare things that will come in handy for one disaster and not another. Do your own research and decide what is most likely to happen. Then gradually begin to purchase the items and equipment that you have decided will be necessary. Naturally, choose the highest quality equipment, because when a disaster breaks out, you'll find that you've actually invested in your life.

4. My rescue kit is tough enough to withstand the tough conditions.

The problem is that if you have a ready-made kit that costs you as much as several beers, you may be unpleasantly surprised. Most survival kit manufacturers source the cheapest equipment of poor quality, as long as the bag has any content.

Your strategy

As with the previous myth, do some research, browse discussion forums, social media, find reviews of the equipment you are interested in. If it turns out that the equipment that meets your requirements is expensive, you don't have to take a bank loan to pay for it. Try to save regularly until you get the full amount. Good quality, reputable equipment is a greater guarantee of security than something that costs little, but when it comes to what will fall apart in your hands.

5. I don't have any clothes in my rescue kit; I'll only have the ones I'm gonna be wearing on the day of the crash.

The problem can happen in an instant. Because what are you gonna do if it's cold and you get soaked to a dry thread? You survive a nuclear explosion and die of pneumonia. Pretty funny, right? Wearing wet clothes in bad weather is a recipe for hypothermia.

Your strategy.

First of all, put your clothes alternately in the bag you're preparing for a disaster. It doesn't have to be a woolen sweater or a down jacket. You'd have to have a big trunk to carry it all with you. I hope I don't have to tell you why a trunk like this is a bad idea? Invest in underwear, light, breathable pants, raincoat, hat, warm socks, boots above the ankle. Modern outdoor clothing is really high quality, and you can have a set of clothes that will weigh as much as nothing and will save your life in a critical moment.

6. I'll just use the phone, so I don't need any alternative communication equipment.

The problem will arise when the telecommunication towers stop working for some reason, for example, by the lack of power. Your situation can quickly turn out to be a little bit uncomfortable if you rely entirely on your phone, and suddenly, the network stops functioning.

Your plan

Signal mirror, flares, walkie-talkie with spare batteries. The mirror can signal your position over several dozen miles. A radio, such as a CB or a walkie-talkie radio, will be most effective if you are in town.

7. A rescue kit is a rescue kit. It's a guarantee that I will survive.

The problem is that you assume that your survival depends on the equipment. You think that if you have the best equipment, nothing bad will happen to you. But I can easily prove you wrong. Because what if the equipment breaks down? What if it breaks?!

Your strategy.

To deal with the problem of broken equipment, you need to work on a strategy for making some kind of backup. For example, if you have battery-operated products, why not buy batteries and a battery charger instead? Do you have solar-powered chargers? What if there is no sun? Do you have an alternative to this type of power supply? Of course, you can count on it indefinitely until it becomes absurd. The point is rather that you are aware that equipment is just equipment and can simply break down.

8. My rescue kit will allow me to wait calmly for the worst anywhere.

The problem is that most people believe they can wait. However, in reality, there is a good chance that you will get involved in a difficult struggle for survival as if there were not enough resources accumulated in one small bag.

Your plan

It's good to have a rescue kit, even very good. But don't ignore the possibilities that will give you your own home. Survival courses, training, trips to difficult terrain with instructors - former commandos give the illusion that I can and do everything, nothing bad will happen to me, and I can stand everything. Meanwhile, my own home may turn out to be crucial for surviving the cataclysm.

Go through these eight misconceptions again and discover what not to do when the next time a disaster happens. Think about this list creatively and consider what other misconceptions you would like to face.

Survival In An Uncertain World.

In today's world, there are several factors that overlap to create synergies:

- Population growth;

- Global warming;

- Environmental pollution;

- Growing demand for food;

- Climate change;

Imagine an overpopulated planet struggling with unpredictable weather events. Fighting for limited resources during the worst economic crisis in history. Many people are expecting disaster and, at the same time, are totally dependent on large corporations guaranteeing technological progress and government institutions.

General Russel L. Honore, the commander in charge of calming the situation after Hurricane Katrina, has suggested with the most important lesson we should learn from this disaster is that humanity should regain its survival instinct. In pre-war society, as Honore claims, Americans made sure that a culture of survival was developed. This culture was characterized by self-sufficiency, independence, and the ability to prepare for the worst. It was common at that time to store food and water for long periods of time, to develop survival skills, to keep machines and equipment in good condition, which at the time of crisis or disaster could significantly improve the safety of individuals and communities.

The loss of the ability to take care of one's own fate and survival instinct, according to General Honore, has led us to a kind of disability manifested by helplessness in times of crisis and an exaggerated faith in government institutions that often fail at critical moments, or their reaction is late. We are now living in times that pose enormous challenges. It is not uncommon for overlapping natural disasters, one hurricane after another, on the scale of Hurricane Katrina, to be accompanied by an economic crisis, unemployment...

All of this puts us to a huge test, and the first thing we should do is start rebuilding the survival instinct that has helped our ancestors repeatedly. We have to stop thinking that "this thing" can happen to someone else. A potential threat (you can recall the current events related to the Coronavirus pandemic) can happen to anyone without exception.

The key to rebuilding the survival instinct is to instill it again in our communities and families. Let's spend at least one weekend a month discussing with the family how to act when a natural disaster, an outbreak of epidemics, or threats of war occurs. Let's discuss a situation in which we can't drive a car, get the necessary supplies in the supermarket, have no access to telecommunication and IT networks. The only thing you can rely on is yourself, your family, and your home. In such a situation, you must be aware that all that can help you to survive is what you have around you in your home. The scenario of being cut off from any possibility of external supply, interrupting the transmission of resources is the most realistic scenario. At such a critical moment, your lifestyle may change dramatically. You will not be able to brush your teeth in the morning because you will not have access to running water. You won't be able to watch a message on the TV in the morning because there will be no electricity supplied to your home. For the same reason you can't call 911, withdraw money from an ATM, you won't have access to your money.

Because you don't have access to the Internet, you don't know what's going on around you. The food in the fridge breaks down because the fridge is not working, and the house is getting colder. Or when you live in the far south, it gets hotter and hotter because your air conditioning is not working.

Going back to the family meeting, sit down, and decide to simulate all the conditions I have indicated above and try to survive one day or weekend in this way. And now try to think/imagine that you have to live through a month, two or six months. How much do you think you can stand without being prepared for this situation at all? One typical day for your family in a situation where you don't have access to all these resources should lead you to quickly understand that you need to stock up on products from 3 basic categories:

- Food and water;

- Medicine and personal hygiene;

- Safety and self-sufficiency;

Providing yourself with access to products from these three categories will greatly increase your chances of surviving a disaster in your own home. If you plan everything well and consider the most likely scenarios, there is a very good chance that you will survive every possible disaster. Let's now take a brief look at each of these categories, also referring to the points I made in the previous chapters.

Food and water

I suggest that you gather enough food and water for your family so that you can survive a minimum of 7 days and preferably 30. Aim for foods with long shelf-life, freeze-dried foods, canned foods such as beans, wheat rice, nuts, etc. There are many companies that specialize in producing this kind of food; you should also consider foods with high energy value, rich in protein and nutrients. An example of such food is energy bars that have all these characteristics. In the case of water, at least 2 gallons of water per day should be provided for each person. This will be water for both drinking and cooking and washing.

Remember that it should be clean and drinkable water. If you find it difficult to prepare a supply of clean water, plan how you will filter and purify the water. There are many tanks on the market dedicated to water storage—also rainwater.

Medicine and hygiene

Maintaining high sanitary standards is a prerequisite for good health. Try to store perishable food in a cool and dark place, ensure you can get rid of waste and contamination. These are aspects that do not give you a headache on a daily basis when it comes to the smooth running of the sewage system, ventilation, and the smooth running of companies that take away waste and refuse.

However, when suddenly all solutions stop working, we notice how important it is to maintain personal hygiene in a situation where there is a potential risk of infection, which can even lead to death when the health service is not working. Try to have a well-stocked first-aid kit at home where you can keep antibiotics, painkillers and fevers, a complete emergency package in case of an injury, and hygienic items such as antibacterial wipes, disinfectants, hygiene wipes, bleach, soaps. If you have young children at home, don't forget diapers, and if necessary, baby care products.

Safety and self-sufficiency

To survive in a situation where there is no mass of access to the facilities offered by today's infrastructure, you need to ask yourself the basic question of what tools, products, and skills you need to live a productive and safe life for at least 30 days without any outside support. Create a checklist and note down all the resources you have access to and the areas you need to complete in terms of:

- Lighting;

- Shelter;

- Heating;

- Power supply;

- Water filtration;

- Communication;

To function as normal as possible and have contact with the outside world as such, you will need:

- Battery-powered radios;

- Cookers and the fuel needed to power them;

- Fans;

- Knives;

- Can openers

- Kitchenware

- Waterproof matches;

- Insulation tape;

- Duct tape

You'll need ropes, hand tools, sawing basic carpentry tools. Of course, you will also need skills to carry out necessary repairs and solve problems related to equipment failures. The list I mentioned will probably look different for families operating in different latitudes, in different climates. It will depend on the type of local development, the qualifications of the family members, their size, and the ability to store products and equipment in the long term.

Water

———

Always keep an eye on the back of your head: when the moment has come when you should act, be aware that the time for preparation is gone forever. In these times, which I mentioned in the previous chapter, a feature that comes to the fore is the ability to anticipate and prevent. It makes sense to simply equip your family with resources that will help them survive potential disasters, cataclysms, wars, or diseases. Perhaps you should think about taking out disaster insurance. Because the risk of such an event is more likely today than ever.

I would now like to focus on the very important aspect of proper water filtration. The provision of drinking water is a basic guarantee of human safety, health, and life. Given our modern lifestyle, in which we consume huge amounts of water, it is difficult to imagine a world where it is not easily accessible, a world in which it ceases to be as we knew it only yesterday. When there is no water flowing from the tap, there is no electricity in the whole area, and there are panic and a state of disorientation among neighbors, we must be able to switch to emergency mode immediately.

Not only can a situation of lack of access to water from the water supply be a threat and a challenge, but also a situation in which you are forced to evacuate and stay in an unknown place and area with no access to drinking water. If you are in the mountains, in the desert or somewhere deep in the forest, if you don't have enough water with you, it can take a really long time before you find a reservoir or a stream. Water in such a situation, even if it doesn't seem too clean and doesn't resemble bottled water from a supermarket, can be consumed by people.

Of course, you have to remember that there can be microbes, bacteria that can cause you to become ill and die as a result. So make sure to boil for at least 20 minutes if possible. Remember that about 60% of the human body consists of water. This size varies depending on the age of the person and their health. An average person needs about 2 liters of water per day to replace body fluids lost due to sweating, fasting, urination, intensive breathing.

Dehydration is a great danger when we are left alone somewhere in an unknown area. It can be accompanied by fatigue, exhaustion, and lead to hypothermia, brain damage, and consequent death. In hot climates, if you do not replenish fluids continuously, dehydration can occur even within an hour. Life without water can be compared to a car that cannot work without fuel. It just won't happen.

The available data indicate that an average man can survive without food for about 30 days. And he can only survive 3-5 days without water under average conditions. So it's easy to deduce that if you get lost somewhere and stay without water for seven days, you'll most likely die.

Worldwide, at least 10 million people die each year from diseases related to lack of water or consumption of polluted water. Unpurified water can be the cause of serious dysentery characterized by diarrhea, fever, and blood traces in feces. Other diseases caused by protozoa, bacteria, and other organisms are cholera, typhus. All of these diseases quickly lead to death if not available for medical care. It is worth mentioning in this context that your determination to survive should be combined with your readiness and ability to filter water.

In a situation of getting lost in the mountains, as I described earlier, the first task that you should set before you is to find water. In the mountains, water is usually trapped between the rocks; it can also be present in basins, at the foot of mountains or cliffs. Of course, you may also come across streams and stagnant places where animals use water. The next step you should take is to bring the water to a state suitable for consumption:

- Cooking is considered to be the best strategy to eliminate dangerous and invisible microorganisms. Two things are needed to boil water: a container that is fireproof and a match or lighter. If you don't have a fireproof container, the best way is to use heating-up stones to boil water when they get hot, move them all into any water container. Stones brought to a high temperature will cause the water to boil. Whichever method you choose to use to boil the water, remember to boil it for at least 20 minutes,

- Water purification by means of sunlight - with this method, you need two things: first and obviously sunlight, so this method will not work on rainy days. The second is a simple, transparent plastic PET (polyethylene terephthalate) bottle. You will be able to consume the water safely if you place it in this plastic bottle and expose it to sunlight for 6 hours. How does it work? Ultraviolet sunlight kills bacteria, viruses, and parasites present in water. This technique has been shown to eliminate 99% of the microorganisms present in the water.

- Water purification tablets - this should be the last, absolutely emergency choice of water purification method. Such tablets are included in sets intended for the army. However, it should be mentioned that the FDA does not authorize this solution. If you ever find yourself in a situation where you can't boil the water, and the sun is hiding behind dark, dense clouds, use the last solution and clean the water with these tablets. Perhaps this will save your life.

But before you start boiling the water, you should first filter it.

It is likely that the water you find will be dirty and full of organic impurities. The first method you can use at this point is to filter the water through your own sock, so it would be good if your sock were cleaner than the water itself. If you don't have access to a clean sock, you can make a basic water filter using tree cork. Use a knife to remove the rectangular bark from the tree. Shape this rectangle into a cone, find a few small stones and throw them inside, then layered filter using moss, grass, sand, and if you have charcoal available from the fire. Pour water into a dish through the cone; the water is then ready for boiling. When the water passes through such a cone, visible dirt and chemical impurities are removed. Invisible to the naked eye, microorganisms will, unfortunately, not be removed during the filtration process. That is why it is so important to boil the water, as indicated above.

As I have already noticed, our bodies need water to live, not enough water in a scenario where you are struggling to survive can quickly cause dehydration, fatigue, hypothermia, brain damage, and finally, death. Methods of water purification are just as important as the way you seek it. Unfiltered, untreated water is completely useless. This is similar to a situation where there is no water at all. If your life is in danger, you will be forced to use such water, because it is a state of higher necessity. Therefore, in order to protect yourself from the lack of access to drinking water, include in your survival kit, a bag in which you have gathered all the necessary things to survive the disaster, including a kit for filtering and boiling water. The ability to carry out the activities described above is a prerequisite for good preparation for surviving extreme situations.

Natural Medicine In A Survival Situation.

If you find yourself in a situation where you do not have access to the necessary medicines, you can easily panic. The good news is that there are alternatives to conventional medicines that can be as effective as those recommended by your doctor. There are numerous natural products that can help you with abrasions, burns, excessive bleeding, and other physical injuries.

This section will show you alternative medicines. However, at this point, I would like to give you a warning. If you are going to spend a few or more days away from civilization and you suffer from cardiovascular diseases, diabetes, epilepsy or any other chronic disease that requires you to take medication every day, the best solution is to go to your doctor. Let him know that you are planning to stay outdoors for a longer time and ask for one or two months' supply of all the medication you are taking. This solution will also work if you don't plan to go anywhere but want to ensure that you have access to your medication when an unforeseen event such as a natural disaster, pandemic, or war occurs.

However, if you are not able to collect the medicines listed above, there are alternative methods that will allow you to survive the crisis. These are herbs and supplements, which in many cases, can be as effective as the medicines you usually take and sometimes even safer than them. I will now discuss some of the medicines and supplements that I think you should have in your home:

- Apple vinegar - contains all the most important minerals, such as potassium, magnesium, calcium, phosphorus, iron, and sulfur. It is a strong antibacterial agent and can be used to treat various ailments, e.g., vinegar is applied to bites, stings or burns to neutralize the poison and reduce swelling and thus reduce mental stress caused by bee attack, insect bites, etc. When given orally, it can help with digestive problems and is very effective in cleansing the blood and digestive system.

*** make sure that you can buy apple vinegar organic, unpasteurized because pasteurized vinegar is devoid of any vitamins, enzymes, and minerals that help with the above-mentioned ailments

Application:

Diabetes mellitus, the effect of vinegar on blood sugar levels, is one of the better-researched health benefits of this substance. Many studies have shown that apple vinegar can help reduce glucose levels, e.g., one 2007 study on 11 people with type II diabetes showed that taking two tablespoons of apple vinegar before bedtime reduces glucose levels in the early morning from 4 to 6%.

Hypertension - potassium contained in apple vinegar can be beneficial both for heart function and blood pressure reduction. Pour two tablespoons of apple vinegar into a glass of clean water, add a spoon of honey to make the drink tastier.

Arthritis - can be a devastating disease as it can cause considerable pain and discomfort. Gout is said to be a disease caused by toxins that are found in the blood and which accumulate in the joints over time and cause the problems indicated above. These deposits can cause disability and serious joint problems that make walking and movement impossible.

Daily consumption of apple vinegar helps to break down and remove these dangerous toxins from the joints and has been shown to significantly reduce swelling and pain. In addition to drinking vinegar with water every day you can also soak the affected areas in hot vinegar water (in the ratio of fields of a glass to 3 glasses of water)

*** Cider vinegar should not be used by allergy sufferers yeast and yeast products

- Organic coconut oil - the health benefits of coconut oil are unlimited. It has been used for thousands of years for everything related to skin hair care, teeth, digestion problems, kidney function, and improvement of metabolic processes. Its beneficial effects on cancer prevention and stress reduction have also been proven.

Coconut oil has antibacterial, antifungal and antioxidant properties, and as we know, all these properties are extremely helpful in the avoidance and treatment of diseases.

Application:

Heart disease - among many people there is a misconception that coconut oil is not suitable for the heart. This belief is due to the fact that coconut oil contains high levels of fats. Nevertheless, coconut oil is actually beneficial to the heart. It consists of about 50% lauric acid, which helps to avoid many heart problems, lower cholesterol levels, and help with hypertension.

The saturated fats present in coconut oil are not harmful, unlike the saturated fats contained in other vegetable oils. Coconut oil also helps to prevent atherosclerosis. Coconut oil is composed of acids that help to maintain a healthy human immune system. These acids have a significant impact on preventing and combating various autoimmune diseases. They also reduce the likelihood of falling ill with ordinary flu.

When coconut oil is applied externally to the skin, we gain a barrier, effectively preventing bacteria and microorganisms from penetrating the skin.

Coconut oil is effective in the fight against the disease due to its antifungal and antibacterial properties. Coconut oil eliminates viruses causing flu, measles, liver diseases, herpes, SARS, etc. It also eliminates germs causing ulcers and infections of the throat, urinary tract, pneumonia, gonorrhea, etc. Coconut oil is also reliable in the fight against fungi and yeasts that cause mycoses, diaper rash, etc.

*** Coconut oil should not be used by persons allergic to its ingredients.

- Colloidal silver - colloidal silver is a liquid suspension of fine silver particles; it has been proven to eliminate numerous bacteria. It was also used as an antibiotic before the 1930s. The FDA approved colloidal silver as a disinfectant for healthcare facilities. Applications:

Antibiotics - before they came into use, many people suffered and died from even minor infections. Although antibiotics are now widely available, it is easy to imagine that we will lose access to them. Then take colloidal silver with its antibiotic properties seriously. A standard antibiotic can kill a dozen or so strains of bacteria and is usually used to eliminate a particular type of germs, which causes the development of antibiotic-resistant strains of bacteria.

Colloidal silver kills about 650 strains of bacteria. It inhibits their development immediately after contact and does not differentiate the bacteria in any way, killing them all in turn.

***Silver allergic people shouldn't use it.

- Garlic - raw garlic may be the best solution, easily available in an emergency. Its bacterial properties and effectiveness in fighting infections are known. It can be used topically to eliminate infections, but it can also be ingested to remove microorganisms from the body.

Here I will list a few applications of garlic, which would be most useful where conventional treatment is not available. Application:

Toothache - crushed raw garlic is applied directly to the sore tooth and gum area. When the garlic comes into contact with diseased tissue, the symptoms of infection are alleviated. A side effect of such treatment will be irritation of the sensitive gum skin. We can accept this minor inconvenience if the infection is eliminated as a result.

Earache - to alleviate the ear pain, all you need to do is to turn over a capsule with liquid garlic and drop a few drops into the sore ear canal. Then lie down on your side for about 10 minutes so that the liquid enters your ear canal. The pain and infection should disappear within a few hours.

Breathing problems - put some cloves of raw garlic in a cotton sock or a bag of other breathable material, lie down and place the bag of garlic close to your head or tie it around your neck. This can help alleviate asthma attacks and al-lergic reactions.

Another method is to slice the garlic and place it in a bowl or pot of boiling water. If you have trouble breathing, stand over steaming water with garlic, lean over and cover your head with a towel. Breathe freely over the steaming water allowing the sulfur compounds contained in garlic to enter the airways and sinuses, helping to remove infections and inflammation.

- Cayenne Pepper - is an herb extracted from chili peppers.

Although most of us think of Cayenne Pepper as a spice used in cooking, the use of this herb goes far beyond the cooking area. It is one of the best commonly available herbs because it works very fast, and this feature makes it essential for emergency situations. Application:

Cardiovascular disease - if the patient has a seizure give him warm water with a mixed teaspoon of pepper Cayenne, it has been proven that this treatment will stop the seizure.

Hemorrhage -Cayenne pepper is a very effective painkiller and can be used directly even to treat the largest wounds and pressure. Its characteristic feature is that it can stop the bleeding. It effectively fights infections and promotes recovery.

Convulsions - traumatic experiences, both mental and physical, can cause shock or even convulsions in some people. Pepper Cayenne can help to balance the psychophysical state of such a person.

*** Cayenne pepper used in combination with caffeine can cause severe pain in some people.

Forging Alliances.

W hen considering leadership and group functioning in the context of an emergency and a struggle for survival, think first about how you work with others in your workplace. Effective group functioning in the workplace is about the fact that the group has its own structure, its own leader who delegates tasks to other members of the group, and all members of the group have a common goal they share.

Although not everyone likes to work in a group and it has the noticeable disadvantage of marginalizing the interest of the individual to the interest of the group, its strengths, among other things, productivity related to teamwork, outweigh its weaknesses. Of course, there may be rifts or conflicts when too many people want to lead the group and not enough to submit to and achieve the goals.

It is natural that there will always be people in the group who will be dissatisfied because they do much more work than the previously established division of tasks in the group. Then disputes and conflicts arise.

All these considerations are important from the point of view of one of the goals we set ourselves in a situation of crisis or natural disaster, which is creating alliances. In fact, your chances of survival will be much greater than if you act alone. It is very difficult to ensure the safety of your family in the area of shelter, food, water, repairing broken equipment, defending against criminals and wildlife.

Then it turns out that it is very difficult to do it all by yourself, and that is why we need alliances with other survivors. Besides, even at the moment of the disaster, we do not lose what distinguishes us from other species, namely the extensive productive teamwork.

Perhaps you remember the scenes from the movies "I am Legend" with Will Smith. The protagonist was so desperate to find other people that he was desperate to talk to a dummy in a shop drowning in tears. By entering into alliances, you won't have to deal with the adversity of fate alone, and that can be crucial to your mental and physical well-being. It can happen that you fall ill or suffer an injury, and it will be very difficult for you to take care of yourself and your family if there are no other people around you.

Other people around us are also needed to look at the difficulties and dangers of another person's perspective, and you may find that the situation is not as bad as you thought it would be. Thanks to the alliance, you can gain from the different strengths of the group members.

The group may have a few hunters who are good at using their weapons, let them be responsible for getting food. Someone else can be a skilled mechanic and take care of the ongoing repairs. There can be many functions in the group; it all depends on the needs and skills of the group members.

You may find that the ability to form an alliance will be crucial for survival, as members of another group may have the things you need and vice versa. In order for such an alliance to work smoothly, you need to develop rules of conduct/guidelines.

You can agree that the group management system can be fully democratic, where each person's voice weighs the same. Decision making is done by voting after listening to each person. Nevertheless, it will be useful to create leadership hierarchies. It is necessary to determine at the very beginning who is to be the leader in order to avoid chaos.

It will be much easier for you to form an alliance with someone who was your friend, a neighbor in the days before the disaster. If you could get along with him, then there is a good chance that you will get along with him now. Working together in a group must be based on the principle of trust and the awareness that we can rely on each and every one of the people with whom we are forming an alliance. It is also good to establish a division of responsibilities. Let everyone know that they have to do what they have to do. And that there is nothing for free because everyone in the group has to work and bring some value to it.

At the same time, listen to yourself, your intuition, which tells you that you should not enter into an alliance with a person. There is a high probability that your intuition is not misleading you. If you feel that you cannot rely on someone in your life, you do not have to justify it. You have the right to protect yourself and your family in a manner consistent with your value system.

Being part of a group also brings with it some risks, and you should keep them in mind. It may not be enough to have common goals for food and safety when faced with differences of opinion and stress in a group of more people. While the group is formed to deal with external problems, it may be that mistakes, aggressive behavior, and particular interests of group members will blow it apart from the inside out.

Moreover, another threat is illness. One member of the group who becomes ill can infect other members of the group quite easily and quickly. Then isolating the sick person, although it may be difficult, will be crucial for the safety of others.

Let's assume that your group is already formed, that you have formed an alliance, but there may be others, more people who will want to join you. Then you have to make a difficult decision whether you have enough food and whether your shelter is big enough to accommodate you all. Always take into account the fact that new people will try by force to take over the leadership in your group or by force to take over your resources.

There will come a time when you start to think that maybe it will be better for you and your loved ones if you break the alliance. This may happen when you notice that you have no benefit from staying in the group. It may also be that your goals and those of other group members are diametrically different.

Make the decision to break the alliance only if you are sure you will find enough food yourself, and you will be able to keep your family safe. The essence of entering an alliance is that it is reasonably safe to lead your family through the toughest days just after the disaster. Once the critical moment is over and you have a good enough understanding of the situation, you can try to break away from the group and go your way.

Resource strategies in difficult times

If you think that your ordinary life puts you in too demanding a task, believe me, it will be even harder after the disaster. You can lose everything you have overnight, and you won't be able to rebuild your property by going to work. Considering that a natural disaster, a nuclear power plant breakdown, a pandemic, or war is accompanied by chaos, you will definitely not know what your tomorrow will look like. Since you don't know how it will all turn out, it is advisable that you develop and have several different resource strategies.

Difficult times require you to innovate and act in a non-standard way; you may have to cross the boundaries of your beliefs and do something you would never do in a so-called normal situation. Think about whether if you experience a disaster and break into a grocery store or a pharmacy in search of food or medicine, it will be stealing. The truth is that the strongest survive. You have to reset your moral system and take what you need before someone else shows up and takes it away.

Consider that you are not alone, other people think the same, they want to survive, and the resources available are limited. You have to do everything to get what you need and not get killed.

Consider the fact that the hours just after the disaster are a time of anarchy. There is no federal government, no service, no national guard, no army. They're in a hurry to organize, even if you don't want it, those hours are the time when everything is allowed. You just can't wait passively for a rescue that doesn't know when it's coming. The same goes for the means of transport. The primary goal is to take you and your family to safety.

Once again, you do what you're forced to do by taking someone else's car to get the hell out of here. You need a large amount of money that you can use in case of a disaster. Remember that the technology on which our civilization is based can stop working in the blink of an eye, which means that your money stored in a bank will no longer be available when banks and ATMs lose power.

Always have a few thousand dollars in cash with you, in different denominations. Of course, don't keep all the cash in one place. Post-crash times are a time when everything changes, it's likely that the money won't have any value, but it's a good idea to have some green notes in your bank because there will always be people who want your money in exchange for their resources.

The longer the chaos lasts, the sooner the money stops being a priority for you and other people. The most important thing is to get food and have a safe haven. If you have valuables such as silver coins, jewelry, or anything of any value like money, you can always meet someone who will be interested in your gold and silver by giving you back your firewood or medicines they have. Even in times when the world is coming to an end, people like to have nice, shiny things. If you have an excess of a certain group of products, you can exchange them for others that you need more.

In difficult times, for example, alcohol can be a new currency and a commodity that people really need. Someone may want to give you your clothes or food for a few bottles of good vodka that you have with you. But be careful when offering weapons in this exchange.

The same goes for ammunition. This type of material will certainly be very difficult to obtain, as you may find yourself in a situation where the person to whom you have given your weapon in exchange for medicine or food will want to take everything you have by force away from you.

Be prepared and alert every day

Being prepared for everything every day is necessary to survive. Of course, this doesn't mean that the real and potential threat in the world after a disaster constantly occupies your thoughts, poisons your life, and eliminates joy. Just be alert and sensitive to the signals coming to you from everywhere.

It was only after September 11, 2001, that many people began to see the need to be on alert. On that day, Americans saw that their country could become a victim of incalculable evil and that their safe everyday life was about to disappear forever. On that day, they did not know if this was a war or a tragic tangle of random events, they were terrified, they did not know where their family was, they did not have any strategy or products in-store.

So far, they believed that nothing bad on their own land could happen to them. They simply changed what they believed in, and now they are ready for anything.

Many people nowadays no longer listen to the daily news. They don't want to listen all the time about disasters, accidents, misfortunes that are happening in the world. However, you must know that when the day of disaster comes, such news will be an extremely valuable source of information about what is happening around you. Just try not to miss out on the fact that something important has happened, and be sure to get the news to you very quickly. Unfortunately, you can't always count on social networking sites, due to a lot of scams and fake news.

Pay attention to the state of the weather, meteorologists are able to predict weather conditions, but their predictions are not always 100% accurate. If you hear about an upcoming storm, try to protect your home as much as possible. Don't underestimate the warnings; just look for shelter. Don't rely solely on weather forecasts, but also watch the sky, nature, pay attention when the temperature drops sharply, or the wind is getting stronger. This can be a prediction of something much more dangerous.

Keep your phone always charged, keep the charge bars at a constant top level, have your phone charger both at home and in the car. You may not be able to charge your phone at a critical moment, but don't rely solely on your phone's memory. Write down the most important numbers on a piece of paper, copy them, and give them to your family. It may happen that the mobile phone network will be very overloaded and you will have to use your landline. Think about it; you don't really know all the phone numbers of your loved ones by heart, always have cash in your wallet in case of an emergency.

As I wrote in the previous section, you are not guaranteed to be able to get to an ATM or bank and withdraw money in case you have to hurry. Always have a few hundred dollars with you, hide the rest in places where you can easily access it.

Always keep your car refueled, do not let the fuel level fall below half the tank. When disaster strikes, everyone will want to refuel their cars at once. There will be huge queues in front of petrol stations; I think you do not want to experience such chaos.

Always be aware of where your family members are currently staying. Your children's schedules, your wives should always hang from you on the fridge. This way, you can easily determine where they are currently staying. Also, try to establish a checkpoint, a place where you will meet in case of a disaster.

Try to get a good idea of the layout of roads, highways in your area. In the event of a disaster, the road you drive to work every day may be congested. Giant traffic jams will cause you to get stuck somewhere on the road. Try to choose an alternative route from time to time to get to work so that you have the choice and chance to reach your destination when events like this occur despite the traffic jams. The GPS system is getting better and better; it used to happen that it led people into the field instead of getting them to their destination. Always have a GPS receiver at hand and use it wisely in an emergency.

Don't wait until you run out of drugs that you take every day; keep them at least a few weeks ahead. This way, you will have your medication, which you will use in case of an accident.

Keep a constant check on your stock, make a periodic inventory, record the products, their number, expiry date, and map their distribution.

Take care of your body every day, exercise regularly, of course; there are many ways not to do this, e.g., you are tired, busy, or just don't like it. However, you should change the way you think and focus on what you can get by being in better physical shape. Improve your habits, eliminate the harmful ones. Work on your interpersonal communication skills. Every day you have to be fully convinced that you have a strategic action plan and know what to do in case something bad happens. If you care about being prepared, it means that you are well fulfilling your role as a family carer and know what to do to save yourself and others.

We've all surely seen the end of the world on TV more than once. Or some of us have played games where the script assumes the need to survive in the world after a disaster. Hypothetical scenarios seemingly unbelievable can become your reality overnight; you have to use your abilities wisely and be ready for anything.

Developing a solid strategy with different starting points, modes of transport, ways to get food and shelter together with training your skills is very important. You can't assume that when the day of the crash comes, the rescue teams will be on-site right away. Survival without food and drink will be very difficult.

How to avoid losing things?

Most of us will admit that she lost a personal item at least once in her life. With limited resources in a survival situation, the last thing you'd want is to lose the things on which your survival may depend. Then it's extremely difficult to remember where the lost item is, or there will be no way to come back for it. It also has a purely material dimension: you wouldn't want to lose a knife or a multitool, for which you paid few dozen Dollars....

Any tool that is lost or destroyed by incompetent use can affect your further survival.

Below you will find tips to help you solve this problem. Of course, it is best to take some preparatory steps while buying and preparing for expeditions or training:

- Buy tools with bright, glossy linings or handles. In the case of flint or lighter, it's about the color of the material they are made of. The best colors are orange, yellow, red, blue, or white. If you have a choice, avoid dark colors, but of course not at the expense of quality. Yes, camouflage colors will make the object blend into the background, but it will also become invisible to you if you drop it at the wrong place and time.

- If your knife or other tool is in dark matt colors, use an orange paracord or duct tape to add a distinctive feature. You will always be able to quickly remove such an extra detail when needed, or you can use it for other purposes.

- If there's a hole at the end of the knife handle for the cable to thread - do it! This will additionally prevent the knife from being lost, for example, while working. For hidden tang knives or compass knives, you can use your home drill to make up the missing hole.

- Duplicate some equipment (e.g., lighter, matches and flint) - carry one with you and the other in your backpack, never together. These are lightweight items, but they often save lives and let you know where you are, or light up the darkness of the night for a moment.

- If the knife in your knife sheath is loose - repair it with hot air for a plastic knife sheath or an extra stitch for a leather knife sheath. The knife must hold firmly in its cover, especially if you wear it on your belt or neck.

How do you protect yourself from losing things? There are a number of ways to keep the chaos around you under control and protect your items from getting lost. Be careful, especially when you are tired, irritated, or cold.

- Put the items in their place. Try to make a habit of always carrying your penknife in the same pocket.

- Fasten your pockets, especially if you have something in them.

- If your knife or lighter is dark, tie it with reflective tape or something bright (even a fragment of your shirt will be good). Then there is a better chance that you will find them.

- Count the items before you go any further. (I know from experience that sometimes just touching your pocket is not enough - once I was one hundred percent sure that I took a lighter with me and it turned out that there was a new pack of chewing gum in my pocket). Such a simple habit will help you to break the bad luck of losing things.

- Watch your belongings, and before you leave the temporary camp or resting place - make sure you have taken everything. You should make a habit of checking the places you leave. Turning around and looking at the ground takes only a moment and can save you a lot of trouble.

- When you've finished your work, don't stick a knife in a tree or leave it on the ground, just put it in your knife sheath, your permanently worn sachet or pocket. This is a simple but effective method.

- Avoid putting small objects on grass or forest litter - it's better to put them on a T-shirt, single-colored bandana, or bag if you have one.

- If you work with a knife at night, light up the workplace - you will avoid getting hurt or losing the tool. If you have to work in the dark, tie a cord from the handle opening around your wrist or hand.

- If you have any cord, tie the most important tool (e.g., flint, flashlight, compass, or multitool) to a belt or other part of your wardrobe - then even if it falls out while running or falling, you will feel that something is hitting your body.

- For things that you have to use intensively or give to others, use a rope with a small snap hook - you will then be able to easily unfasten the object and attach it back.

- If you are in a group and someone asks you to borrow a tool, sometimes it is better to do the activity for that person or to tie the object to his hand. Just because you haven't lost something doesn't mean she won't do it. Ask that after the work is done, this thing be returned to you immediately. Don't forget to check it before you hide it - "Calm down, nothing's chipped" assurances should only make you more vigilant.

- Periodically check the condition of your pockets and the bottom of your backpack, because sometimes a sharp edge can cut the material, causing something (not just small objects) to fall out unnoticed.

Yes, I know that there are also pendants with a beeper attached to the thing we are afraid to lose. However, somehow I can't imagine someone walking around hanging around with such gadgets. I guess it's better to be vigilant and considerate and leave the toys at home.

One last piece of advice: even if you lose something or lose it in another way, consider whether it is worth spending long hours searching, or whether it is better to spend that time looking for a rescue or a way out of oppression. Things can be redeemed, life, or health - no.

How to avoid destroying things?

S oldiers of all armies of the world have a popular saying: "Take care of the equipment, and he'll take care of you." Every tool has been made for some specific purpose. This does not mean that you can't or shouldn't look for alternative uses, especially if your survival depends on it. On the contrary, that's when you have to get up to the heights of your creativity, to set your imagination free. In general, the knife has the greatest potential for use, allowing you to cut, scrape, stab, hit, or split other materials. But every knife, no matter how perfect it is, has its limitations. Quite often, you can hear a hint of how to baton larger pieces of wood to prepare a stock of wood for the fire. The problem is that every knife has its strength, including weak points, and it wasn't designed for that purpose - that's what an axe is for. A saw, including the foldable, handy one, is also very suitable for cutting wood. In fact, however, in a situation of struggle for survival, using a knife may be the only way to get into dry wood, for example.

A knife is a tool designed primarily for cutting, slicing, or pricking. You are using it to undermine or, as a crowbar, can cause irreparable damage. Respect, maintain and replace your equipment when necessary. The life and safety of your entire group depend on it. Check your own tools regularly, as they are more likely to be damaged.

If you carry a firearm in the field, protect it from moisture at all costs. If there is water in the barrel (e.g., from the snow) and you decide to take a shot, you risk damaging the weapon or causing injury.

The carbon steel blade takes on a grey color after use, which does not have the slightest effect on the quality of the blade. The patina makes the knife more resistant to rusting. Carbon steel knives should be washed, wiped and then dried after use.

In summary: to survive, you need to adopt an effective strategy that takes into account the serious limitations on the quantity and quality of your tools. All efforts must be made to manage the modest resources saved from the disaster so that they can be used for survival in difficult conditions. You should be cautious, composure and cautious in this respect.

Conclusion

Unlike cities, the man did not create nature. We are part of nature, which we seem to forget, believing in the achievements of civilization. And perhaps that's why this mystery continues to cause us a natural attraction to nature. The ability to listen to its rhythm is a milestone on the road to knowledge. Communing with the forest during walks, sports, or survival or bushcraft activities calms the mind, revealing new layers of cognition to us. Moreover, our mental performance improves. It allows us to explore our own limits, confront our personal fears, but also to overcome them.

Each of us wants unique experiences in life. Remember, however, that both nature and the urban environment punish the unprepared. Even seemingly simple activities, such as informing your loved ones where you are going and when you will return, recharging your phone's battery, preparing your equipment and clothes or planning, are of great importance.

To act effectively or reduce side effects, we need to want to do this and know how to do it. The success of even those who come into accidental contact with each other is that they can cooperate in difficult and dangerous conditions. The knowledge and skills brought by each of them can determine the survival of the team. The rules of survival are created by those who survive.

Therefore, check at least some of the guidelines in this guide. Adjust them to your circumstances and the tools you have and, when necessary, change your methods flexibly. American people have always been masters of improvisation. Don't give up even in the most difficult moments. Don't be afraid to sacrifice material things to protect your health. Invest in yourself, not just in equipment. This set of skills, when others give up, can save the lives of you and your loved ones.

As you may have noticed, only selected issues are consciously described here. Therefore, I encourage you to continue your self-development, read other professional positions, and take specialist courses (e.g., first aid). After all, education is supposed to change the consciousness of a person, including a child, develop respect for nature, teach appropriate behaviors, and help to solve problems. We are like a package of our accumulated experience. Become a lifesaver of your life, who discovers and tries to understand the world, not just passively he's watching, waiting for help from others. Only a fool is sure of everything; a wise man keeps asking questions.

Remember that no film, game, or book can replace real contact with nature, elements, tools, and an experienced instructor (e.g., survival).

THE END

About the author

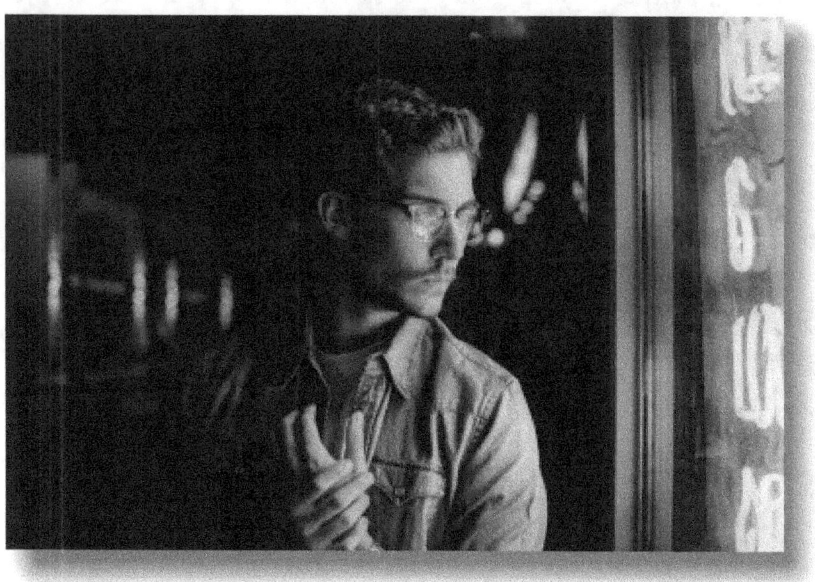

RYAN JONES PH.D. IS a professional career advisor, motivational speaker, and promoter of making changes in life by the method of small steps He is also the author of many books on time management, productivity and habits, and stress management. He graduated from social psychology at the London School of Economics.

His hobbies include personal development, survival and cooking.